THE HAEMORRHAGE CONTROLLER

by

P.S. KAMTHAN

1981

B. JAIN PUBLISHERS
New Delhi-110029

First Edition, 1977
Second Edition, 1981

© *B. Jain Publishers, 1977*

Price : **Rs. 3·00**

Publishers : **B. JAIN PUBLISHERS**
55/I, Arjun Nagar,
New Delhi-110029.

Distributors : **HARJEET & CO.**
1920, Street 10th,
Chuna Mandi, Paharganj,
Post Box 5752, New Delhi-110055.

Printers   : Kapoor Printing Agency, New Delhi-110055.

PREFACE

The book-let facilitates physicians' task of consultation and correct prescribing. In a sense it will prove a *Clinical Treasury*, having contained there in almost all the remedies with characteristic symptoms for bleeding from any part, and with easy prescribing to check haemorrhage promptly.

Allopathy cuts a sorry figure in checking bleeding while the science of Homoeopathy responds favourably and immediately.

Mainpuri (U.P.)   **P.S. Kamthan**
15th Aug., 1977.

CONTENTS

UTERINE HAEMORRHAGE

Sabina 6-30—(*a*) Is of value where the haemorrhage is connected with uterine congestion or inflammation and when the patient robust and florid and flow is bright-red coloured.

—Dr. Hughes

(*b*) Haemorrhage is of *paroxysmal* nature (Erig.), blood being *bright-red mixed with little clots < from least motion*; *pain from sacrum to pubes* (Viscum, Apoc.) *Note* :—Bleeding is less when walking.

Ipec. 1x-3x—(*a*) Dr. Jahr always began with Ipec. and found it magnificent to check red haemorrhage caused by parturition or abortion.

(*b*) One of the most valuable remedies in uterine haemorrhage ; *blood bright red, faintness oppressed breathing and persistent nausea.* **Dr. Cowperthwaite**

(*c*) Dr. Yingling says : "In uterine haemorrhage if Ipecac fails, Pyrogenium is to be given.

Nit. Ac. 6—According to Dr. Hughes, Dr. Claude, Dr. Ludlum and Dr. Amerman endrose the use of Nit. Ac. in prolonged metrorrhagia (*bright red*) which follows abortion or parturition when *mucus lining of uterus is injured.*

Viscum. Alb. 30—(*a*) *Red-clotted* and partly clotted and dark haemorrhage, generally at climacteric period, *with* *pain from sacrum into pelvis radiating downwards*, worse from motion. Dull headache.

Bell. 6-30—(*a*) A most valuable remedy, especially in the post-partum variety, blood bright-red, hot (Lac. C., Puls.), in gushes and cerebral symptoms.   —*Dr. Cowperthwaite*

(*b*) *Frontal headache and hot blood* have always been my guiding symptoms.

Mill.—*Bright-red but non-coagulable* copious haemorrhage, caused by fall (Arn. M.) abortion or parturition.

Erig. 3.—Bright-red haemorrhage of paroxysmal nature (flow comes in sudden gush and stops and re-starts) *with painful micturition* (Mitchel., Thlas.). Often after abortion, sycotic history. (Tereb, Acon, Canth). *Note* :—When Erig fails, Mitchel, performs the task.

Trill. 3x—Active or passive *bright-red* (mostly copious and gushing), sometimes dark and clotted, caused by abortion at or about climacteric period (Arg. N., Aloes., Lach, Sec. C., Sang., Sul., Ust Vinc. M., Viscum.), *with sensation as if hips and back were falling to pieces, better by tight bandage. < on least movement, accompanied by great exhaustion, faintness and dizziness.* (Verat. alb., China., Ferr. M.) *Note* : Cotton absorbed with tincture, if opplied externally, is most helpful to arrest bleeding.

Ustilago 6.—Bright-red haemorrhage—partly fluid and partly clotted, often after parturition, *followed by oozing of dark and clotted blood, from any little over-exertion.*

Cinnamonum φ-3x—An important remedy ; Bright-red haemorrhage cause by *little over-exertion* such as mis-step or over-lifting, often after parturition.

Bovista 30—Bright-red haemorrhage between the menstrual periods (Ambra G., Sab.), often at night and morning.

Note :—Traces of menses between periods from any little exertion—Ambra-G.

Hamm ϕ**-1x**—If haemorrhage is of *dark, non-coagulable, passive and painless nature* Hamm. is the best remedy.

China 3.6.—(*a*) Frequently called for in ante-partum and post-partum haemorrhage. —*Dr. Farrington*

(*b*) Painless, dark-clotted haemorrhage caused by uterine atony, *followed by extreme prostration, faintness and dizziness* wants to be fanned but lightly.

Sec. C. 30-200—(*a*) Extremely useful in uterine haemorrhage from antony of uterus, after parturition or abortion or during climacteric, flow offensive, worse from least motion.

Dr. Cowperthwaite

Note :—Dr. Alley says : "Extremely dangerous when there is Albuminaria".

(*b*) All haemorrhages (from any part) are liquid, *painless dark and offensive*, exited by motion and *accompained by great heat with desire to he uncovered.*

Note :—When this dark haemorrhage is accompanied by *horrible burning, Anth.* is the remedy.

Thlaspi ϕ **1x-6**—Dark clotted haemorrhage accompanied by uterine or lower abdomen *colic* (*crampy or labour-like*—Vib. Op., left sided colic. Canth. Cimic.), aching in back or general bruised soreness, caused by abortion or parturition, uric acid in urine.

Cham. 3-6—(*a*) A very valuable remedy for uterine haemorrhage ; the flow is irregular, dark and clotted.

Dr. Allen

(*b*) *Dark-clotted* haemorrhage caused by parturition or abortion and *attended by severe labour-like pains.*

Crocus. **3x**—*Dark-clotted and stringy,* worse from slightest movements, caused by parturition or abortion.

Caulo 6-30—*Dark-fluid oozing of blood* for days together (Carb. V., Sec. C., Ust., Nit. ac., Ninc. M., Kali C.), after abortion owing to the relaxed condition of blood vessels and want of tonicity.

Platina—Dark-clotted haemorrhage *with spasms, feeling of chilliness* and sensitiveness of parts ; *feeling of constriction and numbness* also appears in certain parts of body.

Elaps 6—Dark. clotted and mostly *fluid blood* (Crot. H., Am. C., Sul. ac.) with or without pain attened generally *by cold feeling in stomach* whereby cold things disagree *i.e.* cause *nausea*, vomiting (Ipec., Apoc.) and general *paralytic condition of limbs*, especially right side.—Feeling of weight in the affected part is a guiding symptom.

Nux. Vom. 6—Dark haemorrhage with *feeling of chilliness and desire* for passing stool.

Aloes 6.30—(*a*) Aloes given in small but frequent doses, deserves to be accounted to be the *best remedy* for those *prostrated, exhausting and obstinate haemorrhages* (especially red) from uterus which occur in women of relaxed nervous and phlegmatic habits about the critical periods of life.

—Dr. Eheriec

(*b*)   *Heaviness and fullness in pelvic region with bearing down feeling in uterus* cannot be neglected as guiding symptoms while prescribing.

Kali C. 30-200—(*a*) Useful in cases of uterine haemorrhage (of constant oozing nature after copious flow) that have been incessant in pale waxy haemorrhagic women, incessant haemorrhage following abortion.

(*b*) *Lumbago* relieved by sitting and pressure and *stiching pains* in lower abdomen accompany almost *every uterine haemorrhage.*

Pyrog.—Dark and offensive haemorrhage in septic states.

Geran. Mac. (30 drops a dose)—Post-partum haemorrhage specially when uterus is badly ulcerated (Kreos., Both., Carb. V., Lach., Nit. ac., Crot., Sul. ac., Phos., Sec. C.)

Vinca Minor 3x—(*a*) I have found it excellent for checking haemorrhage *recurring* some years after climacteric.

—Dr. Hughes

(*b*) *Continuous flow at climacteric period* has often been stopped immediately by me, *great weakness and copious red haemorrhage* were the symptoms. Puls.—Dark clottic intermittent and paroxysmal.

Calendula—I have used the 200th in some cases of bleeding both vaginal and rectal with good results.

—Dr. Stevens

Note :—Haemorrhage from *Cancer or Fibroids*—Calc. C., *Hydr., Mur.*

10

Nit. ac., *Phos.*, *Sab.*, *Sec.*, C., Sil., Sul. ac., Led., Kali. iod., *Kreos.*, *Luch.*, Tereb., *Thlaspi.*, *Trill.*, *Vinc. m.*, *Ust.*, Med., Lapis. A.

Haemorrhage from *Injury—Ambr.*, Arn., *Cinnam.*, Ham., *Mill.*, Sul. ac.

Haemorrhage from *Parturitio1 or Abortion* —Arn., Bell., Caul., Cham., Chin., *Cinnan.*, Croc., Geran., *Erig.*, *Hamm.*, Ipec., Mill, Nit. ac., *Sab. Sec. C.*, *Thlaspi.*, *Trill.*, *Ust.*, Kali C.

Haemorrhage at or about *Climacteric period*—Aloes, *Calc. C.*, Carb. V., Croc, Kali. C., *Erig.*, *Lach.*, Med., Nux. V., Psor., Puls., *Sab.*, Sang., *Sec. C.*, Sep., *Sul.*, Trill., *Ust.*, Arg. M., *Vinc. M.*, *Viscum.*

Haemorrhage from *retained placenta—Bell.*, Canth., Carb. V., *Puls.*, *Sab.*, *Sec. G.*, Sep., Stram.

Haemorrhage in *little girls*+Cina.

Haemorrhage in *Septic fever*—Pyrog., Crotalus.

Haemorrhage as with *convulsions*—Caul., Bell., Hyos., Sec. C., Cimic., Mag. M.

Haemorrhage in *atonic condition of uterus*—Chin., Alet., *Holon.*, Caul.

Haemorrhage in *Paroxysms* —Bell., Cham., Chin., *Erig.*, Nux. V., *Puls Sab.*, *Ust.*, Psor.

Haemorrhage *Continous*—Apoc., Arn., Carb. V., Erig., Cham., Ipec., Kali C., Kreos., Mill., Phos., Sec. C., Sul., Ust. Hamm., Psor., Vinc. M.

Haemorrhage with *painful micturition—Mitchel.*, Thlas., *Erig* : Canths.

Haemorrhage with *labour like pains*—Caul., Cham., Cimic., Vib. op., Hamm., Sab., Sec. C., Thlaspi., Viscum.

Haemorrhage with *pain from Sacrum to Pubes or groin or around pelvis*—Bell., Puls., Sab., Sep., Viscum.

Haemorrhage from *hard stool*—Ambr., Lyc.

Haemorrhage from Sub-involution of Uterus—Alet, Lill. T., Psor., Sec. C., Sel., Sul., Ust.

Haemorrhage *copious*—Arn., *Bell., Calc. C.,* Cham., China., Ipec., Kreos., *Nux V., Phos., Sab., Sec. C.,* Trill., *Mill.,* Nit. ac., *Hamm., Cinnam.,* Caul., *Plat.*

Haemorrhage *Bright-red*—Arn., *Bell.,* Bov., *Calc. C.,* Cham, *Cinnam, Erig.,* Hamm., *Ipec.,* Kali. C., Lac. C., Led., Med., *Mill.,* Mitch. *Phos., Sab.,* Sang., Sec. C., *Trill.,* Ust., Viscum.

Haemorrhage *Bright-red with Clots*—Arn., *Bell.,* Cham., Erig., *Ipec.,* Kali C., *Sab.,* Trill., *Ust.,* Viscum., Cinnam.

Haemorrhage *Dark, Fluid*—Hamm., Sec , C., Elaps., Crot. h., Sul. ac., Am. C., Carb. V., Kreos., Both., Lach., Ars. alb.

Haemorrhage *Dark Clotted*—Cham., *Chin.,* Croc., Cocc. C., Lyco., Puls., Sab., Sec. C., Ust., *Thalsp, Plat.,* Vinc. M.

Haemorrhage *Offensive*—Cham., Croc., Crot. H., Kreos- Sab., Sec. D., Ust., Carb. V., Psor., Lach.

Haemorrhage *Gushing*—Bell., Cham., Chim., Croc., Hamm. Ipec., Mill., Phos., Sab., Sec.. Trill., Ust.

Haemorrhage *Continued but slow*—Carb. V., Hamm., Psor., Sec. C., Sul., Ust.

Haemorrhage *Inter-menstrual*—*Ambr.,* Arg. N., *Bov., Calc. C., Cham.,* Elasp., Hamm., *Ipec.,* Mag. S., *Phos., Sab.,* Vinc. M., Bell., Arn.. Climic., Chin., Croc., Elaps., Kali. C., Lac., Mag. C., Nit. ac., *Rhus tox.,* Sec. C., Sep., *Sil.,* Sul.

Haemorrhage *worse after exertion*—*Ambra.*, *Bov.*, *Calc. C.*, Croc., *Erig.*, *Mill.*, Nit. ac., Rhus. tox., *Trill.*, *Cinnam.*, Hamm., *Bell.*, Cham., *Ipec.*, Mitchel., Phos., *Sab.*, Sec., Ust., Viscum.

Note :—Mangifera Indicaϕ—One of the best general remedies for passive haemorrhage—uterine, renal, gastic pulmonary and intestinal. It compares with Erig. ϕ.

Miscellaneous Haemorrhage (*Bleeding from various other parts*) :

Bovista—Haemorrhage after extraction of teeth, from wounds, epistaxis. —*Dr. Allen*

Arn. **M.**—Bleeding from teeth extraction. —*Dr. Dewey*

Phosphorus—Very useful for a bright-red haemorrhage after tooth extraction. —*Dr. Kent*

Hammmaelis—*Venous* haemorrhage from gums and urine.

Nit. Acid—Excellent remedy for red bleeding from gums, as a result of pyorrhoea (for darkish haemorrhage—Carb. V., Kreos., Hamm.)

Opium—Certainly a great valuable remedy as a palliative in cerebral haemorrhage. —*Dr. Allen*

Note :—Hamm. and Crot. H. are excellent remedies for darkish haemorrhagic measles, sometimes Phos. acts well if the haemorrhage is bright-red.

Alumen—Bleeding after extraction of teeth.

GASTRIC BLEEDING

Ipecac 3x—(*a*) *Bright-red* bleeding with *persistent nausea,* oppressed breathing (Cap. S., Con), *thristlessness.*

(*b*) No better or efficacious remedy.　　　　　—*Dr. Baehr*

Hammamelis 1x—*Dark and thin* bleeding *with feeling of soreness,* pain and throbbing in stomach.

Carb. V. 3-6—Dark and offensive haemorrhage attended by *sensation of great heat-wants to be fanned all the time, rancid belching and extreme prostration.*

Note :—If Carbo V. fails, give Carbon an. or Pyrog.

China 6—*Dark and clotted* haemorrhage followed by extreme prostration, even faintness and attended by *flatulence and aversion to food.*

Crot. hor. 6-30—*Dark or coffee-ground* haemorrhage, cannot retain anything, *vomits everything, faintness and sinking out stomach.*

Ars. alb. 3-50—Dark and thin haemorrhage accompanied by intense heat, thirst—*cold drinks are vomited immediately,* great *anxiety,* and extreme *prostration* to the point of faintness.

Sul. ac. 30-200—Dark haemorrhage (Lach), *accompanied by sour vomiting.*

Sec. Cor. 30-200—*Dark, thin and offensive* haemorrhage accompanied by *intense burning, thirst, nausea and tympany.*

14

Merc. Cor. 6-30—Dark or red haemorrhage, accompanied vomiting *greenish* matter and mucus, *sensitiveness of epigastrium, stomatitis with salivation and night aggravation.*

Pyrog. 30-200—*Dark and very offensive haemorrage,* accompanied by *septic state.*

Trill. 3x—*Bright-red* haemorrage accompained by *heat and burning in stomach,* radiating to oesophagus, *extreme prostration* faintness and buzzing in ears.

Phos. 6—Bright-red or black haemorrhage, *accompanied by great burning which is relieved by cold drinks.*

Cact. G. 6—Bright-red haemorrhage, accompanied by heaviness in stomach, pulsation of palpitation and *tight feeling about chest.*

Vert. alb. 6—Bright red or *black* haemorrage followed by *cold perspiration specially on forehead.*

Ferr. Mur. 6—Dark-clotted haemorrhage (from stomach or lungs), accompained by *anaemia pale face subject to flushes,* pain in right shoulder and elbow.

Hydras. 3x—Haemorrhage of any kind, *from cancer or ulcer* (Geran., Ornith) *in stomach, accompanied by constipation.*

Ficcus Rel. 3x—Bright-red haemorrhage accompanied by *exhaustion* and *restlessness.*

Acet. ac. 6—30—Haemorrhage of any kind, *accompanied by intense burning in stomach radiating to chest, anaemia, oedema of extremities.*

Ornith. 3x—Haemorrhage of any kind from gastric ulcer, accompanied by pain *sometimes after eating and rising of flatus* *in balls here and there.* Dr. Boericke advises single dozes of mother tincture and to wait for action.

Note : (*a*) Vomits blood after fall or injury-*Arn., Mill.,* Ac., Sulph.

  (*b*) Vomits coffee-ground blood—Ars. alb., Cad. S., Crot., Lach., Merc. C., Pyrog., Sec. C.

  (*c*) Vomits blood threatening collapse—Carb. V., Ars. alb., Sec., C., Crot. H., Verat. alb., Chin., Cad. S.

  (*d*) Vomits blood from ulcer or cancer. Acet. ac., Cinnam., Ars. alb., Bell., Cad. S., Carb. V., Hydr. mur., Geran., Kreos., Ornith., Phos., Sec. C., Merc. C., Hamm., Bothrop.

  (*e*) For enterrhagia (haemorrhage from bowels)—Arn. M., Alumen., Cinnam., Cocain., Hamm., Ipec., Plat., Lach., Mur. ac., Nit. ac., Phos., Mill.

Cad. Sulph 3x—*Black* haemmorrage ; from gastric ulcer or cancer, attended by *great prostration, tenderness over stomach persistent vomtting, burning-cutting pain.*

Nux. Vom. 3 x—*Black* haemorrhage, accompanied by *persistent desire to vomit,* weight and pain in stomach, stomach sensitive to pressure and *morning aggravation.*

HAEMORRHAGE FROM BOWELS

Cinnam.-φ-**3**—*Bright-red* haemorrhage from bowels, accompanied by *pain, fetor, flatulence* and sometimes diarrhoea.

Cocaina 3x—Haemorrhage *accompanied by formication and numbness in skin* especially in fore-fingers.

Crot-H.—Darkish bleeding in septic state, may be partly coagulable, skin yellow, while in Elasp. bleeding is entirely fluid.

Note :—Dr. Clarke has stated that Dr. Burnett made brilliant cures by arresting watery bleeding from bowels with Sanguisuga 5, the other haemorrhagic remedies having failed.

Mur. **Ac**. **6-30**—Haemorrhage accompanied by *involuntary stool while passing urine and great prostration.*

Lach. **30-200**—Haemorrhage like *charred straw, black particles, abdomen tympanitic and sensitive to touch,* <after sleep.

Nit. **Ac**. **6**—(*a*) Bright-red haemorrhage from bowels accompanied by *run-down constitution and cutting pains which are worse after stools.*

(*b*) It is one of the best remedies for bleeding from bowels.

—*Dr. Lilienthal*

(*c*) Dr. Bhanja used 200th potency and cured a typhoid case without repetition.

Phos.-6—Bright-red haemorrhage *accompanied by great heat internally with desire for cold drinks.*

Hamm. 1x—(*a*) Dark and thin haemorrhage with *feeling of bruised soreness internally* and sometimes abdominal pain.

(*b*) Where dark venous haemorrhage from the intestines is accompanied with great abdominal pain, it may be Hamamelis. —*Dr. J. Lathord*

Ant. C. 6-30—Copious haemorrhage, *mixed solids of faeces, white coated* tongue and irritabilty of mind.

Ac. Phos. 6-30—Dark haemorrhage with *mental apathy and involuntary stool with flatus.*

Terep. 3x—(*a*) Dark haemorrhage *from ulceration with painful micturition* and red shiny tongue.

(*b*) Haemorrhage from bowels with ulceration, passive dark with ulceration or epithelial degeneration. —*Dr. Allen*

(*c*) Intestinal haemorrhage with extreme tympanitis with red tongue which is smooth, shiny and without papillae, Tereb. is indicated. —*Dr. J. Lathord*

Note :—Red haemorrhage with painful micturition (*Cantharis*).

Nux. Mosch 6-30—*Putrid,* haemorrhage accompanied by *drowsiness, dryness without thirst and rumbling in abdomen.*

Platina. 6-30—*Dark and clotted* haemorrhage (*Am. M.* during menses), *fluid blood mixed with large clots.*

Alumen. 6-200—Has intestinal haemorrhage (for instance in typhoid), with *big clots* and much weakness but without much pain. —*Dr. J. Lathord*

18

Arn. Mont. 3-30—*Arn. M.* and *Mill.* are of service when haemorrhage is due to fall or injury.

Note :—1. One should make a note that above drugs have to be remembered specially while treating *patients of typhoid* if intestinal haemorrhage occurs.

2. According to Dr. Grimmer, *Calend.* , *Succus 200* has sometimes benefited patients stopping haemorrhage and improving malignant and ulcerated conditions both.

3. When haemorrhage is horribly offensive and dark, think of *Pyrog.*, *Ars. alb.* and *Carb. V.*)

HAEMATURIA

(Discharge of blood with urine, either from kidney or bladder)

Cantheris. ϕ.3x-3.6—Haemorrhage either from kidney or bladder accompanied by *bladder irritation, intolerable constant urging to urinate.*

Aconite. 3x—(*a*) *Acon.* is of undoubted efficacy.

—Dr. Hughes

(*b*) When *exposure to dry cold* is the cause, *Acon.* must not fail.

Thlaspi. 1x-6—(*a*) Dr. Hughes makes reference of several eminent physicians and describes it as "easily arresting haemorrhage in general".

(*b*) Nothing equals *Thlaspi* ϕ-3 drops in tea-spoonful every few hours.

—Dr. Guzolar

Ars. Hydr. 3-6—Haemorrhage from kidney *attended by nausea, anaemic conditions, anxiety*, and sometimes suppressed urine and penis covered with eruptions.

Anilin—Haemorrhage as a result of *tumours of the urinary passage* (*Ant., Pyrog*).

Hamm. 1x—*Dark* haemorrhage with passive congestions of kideny and *dull pain in the renal region.*

Tereb 3x—(*a*) Bright-red or dark bloody urine connected with kidney derangement and *painful retention of urine.*

(*b*) Inflammation of kidney with haemorrhage, dark, passive, fetid, strangury with bloody urine.   —*Dr. Boericke*

Nit. Ac. 6-30—Bright-red bloody urine, accompanied by albuminous *offensive urine and cutting pains* ; *urging after urination*, shuddering during urination.

Ficus Rel. 3x—Bright-red bloody urine has once been brought to normal condition by using repeated doses of *Ficus i.e.* every 20 to 30 minutes the guiding symptoms being *uneasiness, and extreme weakness following haemorrhage.*

Milifolium φ—According to Dr. W. A. Davidson, London, *Mill.* is one of the best remedies for haematuria, he cured all the cases within 4 or 5 days.

Erigeron φ-3x—Generally red bloody haemorrhage from bladder with painful micturition (*Mitch., Tereb, Acon., Canth., Thlaspi*), the *flow always being paroxysmal.*

Ipec—(*a*) Excellent remedy in haematuria.

—*Dr. Farrington*

(*b*) I prescribe it successfully if nausea and bright-red bleeding are present.

Coccus Cacti—Large black clotted haemorrhage from kidney comes under the influence of *Cocc. C.*

HAEMORRHOIDAL HAEMORRHAGE

(*Bleeding from Piles*)

Collinsonia ϕ—*Reddish haemorrhage* is checked in majority of cases, if *Collin.* ϕ in 10-drop doses is used thrice a day.

Note :—Patients with tendency to chronic constipation and threatening the appearance of piles are benefited.

Hamamelis ϕ-**1x**—(*a*) *Darkish, non-coagulable, copious* and painless haemorrhage with feeling of soreness in rectum.

(*b*) The most effective remedy both externally and internally for bleeding haemorrhoids.   —*Dr. Cowperthwaite*

Millifolium ϕ—Reddish, non-coagulable, copious and painless haemorrhage has been easily put to check many times by the use of mother tincture in 10-drop doses thrice a day.

Ficus Rel. 3x—Cures haemorrhages of many kinds—Haematemesis. Metrorrhagia haemoptysis.   —*Dr. Boericke*

Kali. C. 30—Reddish copious haemorrhage accompanied by *back-ache, burning-stitching pain and sensitiveness to touch.*

Aesculus 30 —*Haemorrhage accompanied by back-ache affecting sacrum and hips, aggravated by walking and stooping,* rectum is often felt as if full of sticks (Collin).

Sabina 30—Haemorrhage copious and bright-red, *accompanied by pain from back to pubes.*

Ammonium C. 6-30—Haemorrhage during menses.

Capsicum 6—*Haemorrhage with soreness* (Hamm.), *heat and construction.*

Erigeron φ-3—Haemorrhage *with painful micturition* (Thlaspi, Canth., Mitch., Tereb., Acon.).

Nitric Ac. 6—Bright-red haemorrhage with stitching pain in rectum.

Phosphorus 6—Bright-red haemorrhage *with feeling of heat internally and desire for cold drinks.*

Thlaspi 1x-6—Bright-red haemorrhage with *bruised feeling over the body and urinary disorders.*

Nux Vom.—Sometimes haemorrhoidal bleeding is magically stopped by Nux., if constant urging to stool (Aloe., Sep.) is present.

Note :—1. Haemorrhoids that bleed easily, Puls. acts best in higher potencies after Aesc. *Dr. Dewey*

2. Dr. Burt says that no remedy can equal Collin. in obstinate cases of haemorrhoids which bleed almost incessantly, to be given in mother tincture.

3. Dr. Hughes esteems this (Ham.) remedy as one of the best remedies in bleeding piles, recommending the use internally in 2nd dilution and the tincture externally.

4. Ferr. ph., if alternated with Cal. fl., every $\frac{1}{2}$ or 1 hour easily controls bleeding from piles.

5. Sometimes when other drugs fail, Sul. 30, morning and Nux. V. 30 twice (evening and night) daily, serve the purpose.

6. Dr. Boericke has referred Acalypha in rectal haemorrhage in morning.

7. Dr. Stevens has checked rectal bleeding by using Calendula 200, while Dr. Woodburg has emphasised the application of Calendula locally in potency.

8. Drugs indicated in haemorrhage from any part of the human body—Carb. V., Ferr. Met., Melil., Sec. C., Trill., Cinnam., Thlaspi, Tereb., Ipec., Bell., Acon., Hamm., Anthrax., Mill., Ferr. Phos., China., Canth., Crot. H., Croc., Arn. M., Ficus., Calend., Plat., Sul. Ac., Acel. Ac., Kreos., Phos.

9. Bright-red bleeding from piles associated with pain in small of back, extending from sacrum to pubes, is sometimes magically stopped by Sabina 30.

———

EPISTAXIS

(Bleeding from Nose)

Ferr. Met. 30—(*a*) Much confidence in current epistaxis.

—Dr. Cooper, Dr. Hughes

(*b*) Nose-bleed in *anaemic persons* generally, nose is sometimes continually filled with clotted blood ; *face pale but flushed on slightest provocation*, blood being *bright-red mixed with cogula.*

Carb Veg. 30-200—(*a*) Dr. Thays speaks highly of it in epistaxis.

(*b*) Bleeding occurs almost daily accompanied by *pale face and aggravation from slightest strain or exertion.*

(*c*) Dr. Dewey recommends three remedies for *habitual* epistaxis (Ars. alb., China., Carb. V.)

Note :—When Carb. V. fails in checking dark-bleeding, Sec. C. takes place.

Belladonna 6-30—I have used it with success in *warm bleeding* from nose, when coryza is neglected or when the discharge is mixed with blood ; dryness *flushed face and dull frontal headache* often accompany.

Melilotus 6.30—(*a*) Nose-bleed accompanied by *throbbing frontal headache, flushed face and dryness* must breathe through mouth, *headache is relieved by blood-discharge.*

(*b*) *Very red face* precedes haemorrhage from any organ, and affords relief in epistaxis (Bufo., Ferr.ph., Mag. S.)

—Dr. Allen

Erechthites ϕ—Nose-bleed, haemorrhage from any part specially from nose and lungs in *anaemic persons with dropsical swelling of extremities and flashes of heat alternated with coldness.*

Milifolium ϕ—Nose-bleed as a result of injury (Arn. M. which is also one of the best remedies for nose-bleed)—*fall or overlifting, blood being bright-red but non-coagulable* (Carb. V., Crot., Hamm, Phos., Thlaspi., Trill.).

Note :—Mill. or Arn. M. in mother tincture may be applied externally also in distilled water.

Trill. ϕ-3x—Nose-bleed incessant and copious followed by *extreme prostration resulting in faintness, blurred vision and ringing* in ears (China), blood being bright-red or dark-clotted. *Note* :—Dr. Carrier has strongly recommended it for epistaxis.

Thlaspi 1x-6—Nose-bleed in *passive form*, blood being dark, suits patients when urine is loaded *with uric acid or albumen.*

Bryonia—Frequent bleeding of nose when menstruation should appear, also in the morning relieving headache.

—Dr. Boericke

Bovista—Epistaxis specially in the morning after awaking or during night when asleep.

Pulsatilla—Epistaxis during menstrual period, with suppressed menses, bleeding dark, thick, clotted, almost black venous blood.

—Dr. Kent

Hamamelis ϕ·**1x or 30 sometimes**—Nose-bleed, blood being *non-coagulable* accompanied by *bad odour from nose and tightness in bridge of nose.*

Note :—A few drops of Hamm. 1x in a wine-glassful of water and a dose of a tea-spoonful every 5 minutes will do well.

Phosphorus 6—Nose-bleed instead of menses (Bry., Puls., Graph, Lach.) or with chronic catarrh or from polypus (Calc. C., Sang. C.) ; *feeling of heat internally with desire for cold drinks* is the guiding symptom.

Ferr. Phos 1x—Dr. Hughes says : "Ferr. phos. as long ago recommended by Dr. Copper, has often served my turn and never disappointed me."

Mers. Sol. 6—(*a*) Nose-bleed, blood being dark and clotted-blood hangs down the nose like a long black string (Croc., Kali. Bic.)

(*b*) Epistaxis when coughing (Bell., Phos., Arn.) at night during sleep, blood hangs in a dark clotted string from nose like an icicle. —*Dr. Allen*

THERAPEUTIC HINTS FOR PARTICULAR AND PECULIAR TYPES OF NOSE-BLEED

1. Nose-bleed accompanied by much sneezing (Lach. nostrils sensitive—Ac. Mur., Bov., Con., Ind., Rumex., Ambrosia).

2. Nose-bleed accompanied by nasal ulceration and stitching pain (Nit. Ac.).

3. Nose-bleed accompanied by feverishness and anxiety but of recent origin (Acon.).

4. Nose-bleed accompanied by painful and burning urination (Canth.).

5. Nose-bleed accompanied by throbbing of heat (Cact. G.).

6. Nose-bleed accompanied by nausea (Ipec.).

7. Nose-bleed accompanied by worms (Cina.).

8. Nose-bleed accompanied by whooping cough (Arn., Bry., Cina., Cor-R. Crot., Dros., Ipec., Led., Merc., Mur. ac., Nux. V.).

9. Nose-bleed after a bath or wetting (Calc. S., Dulc., Puls., Rhus. tox.).

10. Nose-bleed during sleep (Bry., Merc., Nit. ac., Nux. V., Puls., Sul., Verat. alb.).

11. Nose-bleed while straining at stool (Carb. V., Coff., Phos, Rhus. tox.).

12. Nose-bleed while walking (Elaps.).

13. Nose-bleed from washing face (Am. C., Arn. M., Calc. S., Kali. bic., Kali. C., Tarent., Mag. C.).

14. Nose-bleed in drunkards (Led., Op., Lach., Carb. V.).

15. Nose-bleed in the morning (Nux. V., Nit. ac., Sul., Amb., Bov., Carb. an., Bry.).

16. Nose-bleed in the evening (Ant. C., Carb. S., Lyc., Lach., Sul., Phos. ac., Phos.).

17. Nose-bleed in the night (Ars. alb., Bov., Carb. V., Merc., Nit. ac., Rhus tox.).

18. Nose-bleed occurs between the menstrual period—either at night or early morning (Bov.).

19. (a) Nose-bleed before menses (Lach., Puls., Sul., Verat. alb.).

    (b) Nose-bleed during menses (Amb., Bry, Puls., Sep., Sul., Nat. S.).

    (c) Nose-bleed after menses (Sul.).

20. Nose-bleed after suppressed menses (Bry., Cact., Con.,
Croc., Gels., Lach., Phos., Puls, Sab., Sep.).

21. (*a*) Nose-bleed from right nostril (Bry., Calc. C., Con.,
Cup., Ind., Kali. bic., Kali. C., Kali chir., Mag. C.,
Verat. alb.).

(*b*) Nose-bleed from left nostril (Am. M., Amyl., Berb.,
Caust., Dios., Merc., Rhod., Tarent.).

22. (*a*) Nose-bleed of dark black colour (*Carb. V.*, *Croc.*,
Lach., Elaps., *Nux. V.*, Sec., *Crot. H.*, Ham., Sul. ac.,
Cham., Carb. S., Kali. bi, Kali. N., Merc., Tarent.).

(*b*) Nose-bleed of dark thin colour (*Carb. V.*, *Crot. H.*,
Ham., Lach., *Sec.*, Sul. ac., Ars. alb.).

(*c*) Nose-bleed either black or red (Nit. ac., Lach., Chin.,
Elaps., Kreos., Nux. M., Phos. ac., Puls., Sul., Am.,
Ham.).

(*d*) Nose-bleed clotted (*Bell.*, Carb. S., *Cham.*, *China.*,
Elaps., Croc., Fetr. Ph. M., *Ipec.*, Merc., Nit. ac.,
Phos., *Plat.*, Puls, *Rhus. T.*, Sec., Sul. Tarent., Tub.).

(*e*) Nose-bleed bright red (Acon, Bell., *Carb. ac.*, Erig.,
Cinnam., *Ferr. Ph.*, *Hyos.*, *Ipec.*, Mill., *Phos.*, Rhus.T.,
Sab., Tub.).

(*f*) Nose-bleed offensive (Sec. C., Carb. V., Crot. H.).

23. My mother-in-law who was often a victim of nose-bleed
had once an occasion to bleed profusely and incessantly
in my presence in 1935, the nasal haemorrhage being of
exhausting nature. When one drop of *Carb. V. 200* in an
ounce of water was administered in tea-spoonful doses
every few minutes an immediate relief and check for ever
was the result.

24. Not one but many cases of nose-bleed have been given prompt relief by the use of *Ham φ 1x.* internally and *Ham. φ* externally, no matter whether the blood was dark but non-coagulable.

25. Morning nose-bleed often yields to *Bry.* if headache, thirst and constipation are present.

26. *China* 3x to 30 has become a routine remedy in my hand to remove anaemia or debility following persistent nose-bleed.

27. If *red* haemorrhage *comes on suddenly and from slightest cause* such as over-lifting exertion, etc. from nose, bowels, lungs, uterus, *Cinnam.* 3x in repeated doses will do.

28. Dr. Das Gupta has taken advantage of *Verit. alb.* by checking bleeding from nose (r. nostril) specially at night during sleep with cold body and deathly pale face.

29. Nose-bleed is in itself a key-note of the remedy (Arnica).
—*Dr. Bhanja*

30. Epistaxis when washing the face (Arn., Mag. C.) and hands in the morning from left nostril after eating (Am. C.)
—*Dr. Allen*

31. *Lac. acid*—nose-bleed every morning.

32. *Cros. S.*—black, tenacious and *stringy* with cold sweat on forehead.

33. *Merc. cyan.* 30—This remedy's action in 30th potency is marvellous in checking nose-bleed in diphtheria in children.

34. Aggravation at night—Carb. V., Rhus. tox., Nit. ac.

HAEMOPTYSIS

(*Bleeding from Lungs*)

Millifolium φ--The two medicines on which I have learnt to rely are *Mill.* and *Hamm.* The former is most suitable when the *blood is florid* (bright-red) *and frothy* ; *Hamm.* when the flow is more *pressive and like that of venous* (*dark haemorrhage* : with *neither there is much cough.* —*Dr. Hughes*

Note :—1.   When patient vomits bright-red blood preceded by a *feeling of tickling in chest behind sternum Ferr. acet.* is the remedy.

2.   Dr. Jousset and Dr. Drury have praised *Led.* for *copious vomiting of bright-red blood.*

3.   *Mill.* is the most useful remedy, if haemoptysis is *of traumatic origin* (Arn.).

Calc. Fl.—Calc. fl., if alternated with Ferr. ph., is sometimes of great service in bright-red haemoptysis.

Ferr. Met. 6-30 —(*a*) Frequently a valuable remedy in haemotysis occurring in phthisis, especially in young people who are in the incipent stage of phthisis florida ; flying pains in the chest. —*Dr. Cowperthwaite*

(*b*) Extremely useful when the chest symptoms seem to form a kind of surging of blood to chest. —*Dr. Allen*

(*c*) Haemoptysis on coughing, worse in morning and night, generally in young persons who have indulged in *self-pollution and flush easily.*

Acalypha Ind. φ6—(*a*) Bloody expectoration *preceded by cough, bright-red in the morning* (Kali. bic.) and dark clotted in the afternoon ; feeling of heat from stomach to pyarynx (Phos) ; generally < *in morning* and at night.

(*b*) Most useful remedy in phthisis and haemorrhage from the lungs. —*Dr. Kent*

Geran. Mac. ϕ-3x—Vomits *bright-red blood in large quantity* either from the lungs or stomach ; 10 drops of the mother tincture thrice have several times checked haemorrhage in my hand.

Erecht. ϕ—Stops haemorrhage from lungs accompanied by *scanty urine and swelling of lower extremities*, sometimes flashes of heat alternating with coldness.

Ipecac 3x—(*a*) Holds a high rank. —*Dr. Burt*

(*b*) Ipec. is sure to stop pulmonary haemorrhage if *nausea, oppressed breathing and cough* are present.

Opium 6—Haemoptysis in drunkard, calls for Op. when the *chest is hot and limbs cold.* —*Dr. Farrington*

Calc. Ars. 6—According to Dr. Nankivel, it is useful in bloody expectoration in phthisical patients after pneumonia.

Sticta. P. 3x—In phthisical patients when *persistent, dry, hacking cough* is followed by bloody expectoration and is < *at night*, Sticta. P. helps a great deal.

Kali Nit.—Dry *morning cough* with pain in chest and bloody expectoration, dyspnoea-pulmonary or cardiac, < *morning*, better drinking sips of water.

Phosphorus 6-30 or a single dose of 200—Suits most *tall, slender or rapidly growing persons* who are victims of either pneumonia or phthisis accompanied by *teasing cough with bloody or blood-streaked expectoration* < *in the evening till midnight ; feeling of heat internally with desire for cold drinks.*

Rhus. Tox 6-30—Bright-red and coagulated (dark and clotted—Cham.) expectoration *caused by over-exertion* (Arn.

Ferr,, Mill., Phos., Urt. U.) or difficult and troublesome *cough midnight till morning ; attended by body-aching and restlessness at night.*

Trill. 3x—Red-bloody expectoration, preceded by cough in phthisis *and followed by great prostration —faintless and buzzing in ears* (Chin) is sometimes magically removed.

Cact. C. 3x-6—(*a*) In any haemorrhage seeming to be in any sympathy with heart trouble, think of Cact.   —*Dr. Nash*

(*b*) *Cardiac trouble*—(specially palpitation) along with feeling of bandage about chest are the leading symptoms to prescribe Cact. to stop red-bleeding from lungs.

Note :—(a) Bleeding from lungs threatening collapse—Carb. V., China., Trill., Cact. G., Dig., Crot. H., Carb. an.

(*b*) *Bleeding from lung during menapause* (Lach.).

(*c*) *Bleeding from lungs after suppression of menses* (Acon., Bell,, Bry., Dig., Ferr., Hamm., Mill. Phos., *Puls.,* Sang., *Senec.,* Sep., Sul. ; Ust.).

(*d*) *Bleeding from lungs after suppression of haemorrhoids* [(Acon., Carb. V., Mez., Led., Lyc., *Nux. V.,* Op.).

(*e*) *Bleeding from lungs in drunkards* (Ars. alb., Hyos, Led., Acon, Cavbe. V., Mez., Lyco., Nux. V., Op.).

2. *Profuse bleeding from lungs* (*Arn., Bell.* Crot. H., Caet, G., Carb. V., China, Erecht., Ferr. ph., Ferr. met., *Ferr. acet., Geran., Ham.,* Ipde., *Mill.,* Phos., Sabina.

3. (*a*) *Blood bright-red* (Acal., Acon., Cact., Ferr. met., Erecht., Ferr. ph., acet., Geran, Led., Mill., Nit. ac., Rhus. T., Trill.).

(*b*) *Blood dark clotted* (Arn., Crot., Elaps., China., *Ferr.. Mur.*, *Ham.*, Kreos., *Cham.*, Sec. C., Sul. ac., Carb. ac.).

(*c*) *Bloody frothy* (Acon., Arn., Ferr., Ipec., Dros., Led., Mill, Op., Phos. ac., Phos., Sec., Sil.).

(*d*) *Blood hot* (Acon., *Bell* , Cham., Mill., Bov.).

Kali bic.—(*a*) Most useful remedy for haemorrhage from lungs and phthisis. —*Dr. Kent*

(*b*) *Yellowish string expectoration and morning aggravation* must be the key-symptoms to prescribe.

Kali. iod—Haemorrhage from lungs in syphilitic patients.

Note :—May be used in bleeding from nose, rectum and uterus the history being syphilitic.